The
$A^l_{to} Z$heimer's
Caregiver's
Handbook

Written By
One Caregiver
for Another

Mark A. Nutting

Paperback & eBook available on Amazon.com

ISBN: 9781711870427

Dedication

In loving memory of my mother, who remains forever in my heart

. . . and to her sister, my Aunt Ellie, whose dedicated support and backup in caring for Mom kept me from falling in times when I could no longer stand alone.

RIP Auntie Ellie, Luv, Luv

" . . . *Inasmuch as ye have done it unto one of the least of these my brethren, ye have done it unto me.*"

— Matt 25:40 (KJV)

Disclaimer

The information provided in this book is designed to provide helpful information on the subjects discussed. This book is not meant to be used, nor should it be used, to diagnose or treat any medical condition. For diagnosis or treatment of any medical problem, consult your physician. This book is not meant to be used, nor should it be used, to make legal decisions or create legal documents. For legal issues, questions and documents, consult an attorney for your jurisdiction.

"It is not how much you do, but how much love you put in the doing." — Mother Teresa

Topic Guide

Preface .... *ix*

1 The Early Warning Signs 1

2 The Early Years Of Alzheimer's 7
   a) Early Diagnosis... 7
   b) Treatment... 9
   c) First Lifestyle Changes 10

3 The Ongoing Progression 13
   a) A Few More Changes 13
   b) How Much Is Too Much?.. 14
   c) When It's Gone Too Far 15

4 When They Can't Live At Home Any Longer 18
   a) Proactive Or Emergency?.. 19
   b) The Terrible *Too's* 19
   c) Do You Have The Legal Authority? 21
   d) Selecting A Facility 22
   e) Helping Your Loved One Settle In... 24
   f) Augmenting Facility Care.. 26
   g) Managing Medications in the Facility 29

5 Interacting With Your Loved One As The Alzheimer's Progresses ..32
   a) Redefining Your Relationship 32
   b) Recreating Activities... 33
   c) White Lies... 37
   d) Dolls, Flex Straws, And Mittens... 39
   e) They Often Understand More Than They Can Express 44
   f) And Sometimes They Don't 45
   g) No Credit, Just Love 46
   h) Love And Enjoy Them As They Are 49

6 Medical and Legal Issues 50
   a) Health Care Proxy, Power of Attorney, And Activation 50
   b) Social Security Representative Payee 53
   c) DNRs And Advanced Directives (*Making The Tough Decisions*) . 55

7 Interacting With The Facility 62

8 When And How The End Comes..65
   a) The Last Days and Your Loved One.. 66
   b) The Last Days and You 69

9 Grieving..71

Epilogue: *Caring for the Caregiver*..75

"[Love] bears all things, believes all things, hopes all things, endures all things."

— 1COR 13:7 (KJV)

Preface

The intent of this book is to be a small, quick reference handbook for the primary caregiver of a dementia patient. It is written to relay the issues I encountered as a primary caregiver, and when applicable, solutions that worked for my mother and me throughout her 13-year struggle with Alzheimer's disease. It is intentionally not meant to be an exhaustive or scientific study of dementia or Alzheimer's, but rather a concise reference that deals with everyday life issues I faced when caring for my mother, first in her home, and then in a nursing home facility.

One of my problems when researching Alzheimer's progression and care issues after my mother was diagnosed was that there is an endless amount of information available to sift through. I rarely looked at a book because when I did, they were so involved and in such detail, it always seemed I would have to read through most or all of a several-hundred-page book to find suggestions on the one issue I was concerned with at that moment. When I did find the situation or suggestion I was looking for, often it was a very textbook, medical, or scientific perspective that did not touch our everyday reality.

I've laid out this handbook by topic and subtopic, so it can be used only as a quick lookup when needed, or after reading it in its entirety, as a reference guide.

I am an average caregiver with neither a medical nor a legal background. The medical and legal examples and suggestions I offer in this book are my personal experiences and opinions and are not meant to replace professional medical or legal advice.

1 The Early Warning Signs

Symptoms peaked at the end of 2003, prompting me to schedule a medical evaluation on my mother's behalf regarding her memory changes. But let me turn back the clock a little and discuss some notable changes in my mother's behavior prior to this time.

Whether all of the following items are directly related to or a precursor to Alzheimer's, I don't know, as the doctors did not know. However, the following table is a chronology I compiled for our first diagnostic appointment in January 2004, showing all the memory issues my mother had.

1/19/2004 by: Mark A. Nutting (son)	History of Memory Observations for Carmella A. Nutting
December 1994	Carmella had an episode where she completely forgot common phone numbers, her Social Security number, etc. It took her many attempts of frantically searching to finally find my phone number and call me. I took her to the emergency room and they concurred that there was a memory issue. They kept her overnight and ran some tests. At that time there had been a problem with her furnace and we thought this might be a carbon monoxide issue. However, her blood showed none. I had the house tested and it was fine. I had the furnace replaced just in case. She was fine the next morning and released from the hospital. The diagnosis was "possible hysterical memory loss."

About 1999	Carmella had expressed interest many times about seeing the play *CATS*, based upon commercials and excerpts she kept seeing on television. A couple of months after her repeated expression of interest, I purchased tickets for the show for Mother's Day. Upon receiving the tickets she said she had never heard of that play before. Even once I described (in her words) the details of what she had seen and liked on television she said that I must have her confused with someone else. In a pseudo-acknowledgment that she may have forgotten, and in keeping with her sense of humor, she said, "Well, if I liked it once, I'm sure I'll like it again."
About 2002	Carmella experienced a notable memory loss for a week or two on two or three separate occasions, probably months apart. During these short times, she would have a notable, albeit positive, personality shift (as described below in December 2003).

By the time I would begin to become concerned, she would bounce right back to normal, both in memory and personality. |
| 2002-2003 | Carmella's memory loss appeared minimal and what I had considered normal aging memory loss most of the time. She would occasionally grasp for a word, or forget a recent piece of information (e.g. such as something said in a conversation) – not much different than most people at any age. |
| 2003 | Carmella added an incorrect and inappropriate ingredient (grated cheese) to her beef stew. She has made her same signature beef stew for 50 years and has never put that in before. When told it did not belong in there, she believed she always had put it in. Grated cheese is a very common |

	ingredient she puts in other life-long recipes such as her tomato sauce.
November/December 2003	I began to notice a definite change in the types of memory problems Carmella was having. First, grasping for words and misusing others had increased notably and with more common words (e.g. "pan"). Her favorite restaurant to be taken to for lunch, the Country Buffet, became the "Country Bouquet." Now, after pausing while trying to say it, it is "that Country place". In addition to forgetting short term information, I noticed that she has forgotten older and larger pieces of information — for instance, an entire trip that was taken years ago and a play she attended and enjoyed. Even when reminded and told about the details she still does not remember any part of these events. Also, her ability to learn and retain new information (or relearn forgotten information) seems to be lost or greatly impaired. For instance, she has been having trouble using her headlights because she is confused between how the regular lights and high beams turn on and off. I spent about 15 minutes with her in the car showing her and had her repeat the process several times, but she simply didn't grasp it. When discussing simple things such as scheduling an appointment, she will often just look very confused. Even if the information is repeated many times she will still be unsure of it. Another thing I have noticed over the past year, but more so these past few months, is that she is afraid more — not of anything specific, but just in general.

	Finally, what she refers to as "hearing voices" has been happening for a couple of months. I questioned her about this and she does not hear audible voices, but rather, says arbitrary words will occasionally pop into her head when she is quiet. The example she gave is that while quietly fixing her hair, the word "astronaut" may pop into her head when she was not thinking about anything along those lines.
December 2003	A notable personality shift. Carmella has always been very high strung and nervous. Also, what I would call being depressed for the past 15 years. The smallest problems set her off and she became very excited with crying and overreaction. Now, she is more pleasant, takes things in stride, and what once would have been a major catastrophe to her (e.g. her water pipes freezing) is now treated as a minor inconvenience and almost as an adventure. While the personality shift is positive for many reasons, it is definitely a notable change. I have also noticed a more child-like (not childish) attitude; for instance, a child-like excitement over being taken to lunch, or over a small clock that she just purchased.
Other Current Observations	Carmella still does many things well. She cooks daily (not just for herself, but also for others). I have not seen anything to give me concern about using the stove, etc. Other than the one or two occasions mentioned above, she continues to properly prepare her familiar dishes. She keeps both herself and her home clean and neat and dresses appropriately for the time of day and weather.

	I continue to have her write her own checks and, from balancing her checkbook each month, I can see that she still does well with the math. However, I have noticed a slight decline and more confusion in the checkbook register and writing of the checks over the past two months.
	She still drives, but has restricted herself to day driving only. Also, I've noticed that she does not drive further than probably a five to seven mile radius now and only goes out a couple of times a week. Only a few months ago she was out daily and would go much further. I (or others) now take her on most errands and appointments that go beyond that small radius.
	One other observation that might be important is most of the time Carmella recognizes she is having memory problems and is concerned about it.

I included the above history to show that not all dementia/Alzheimer's cases are *textbook*. My mother's symptoms were not all classic symptoms of Alzheimer's disease. Early on (1994-1999), we thought there might be the possibility of mini-strokes since the incidents were infrequent and she seemed to fully recover from them in short order. Even the drastic one to two week changes that occurred in 2002 seemed to suggest that. However, no diagnosis for those incidents (either showing that they were related to mini-strokes, Alzheimer's, or something else) was given.

The 2002-2003 and 2003 symptoms begin to sound like what I would consider the more common early warning signs of Alzheimer's disease. However, since early symptoms of the disease are easily passed off as normal aging forgetfulness (which is what I did), some of these conclusions are in hindsight.

Certainly, November/December 2003 clearly showed there was a problem more than normal aging forgetfulness. Additionally, it was thought that due to the auditory hallucinations, there might be a Lewy Body Disease (LBD) component and/or mini-strokes because of the personality shift. However, my mother never presented with any other LBD symptoms, and mini-strokes were never confirmed nor ruled out. As you can see, it is possible to have more than one cause contributing to dementia symptoms. In my mother's case, no other causes were ever confirmed, and the diagnosis remained dementia. Since Alzheimer's disease could only be truly diagnosed post mortem via autopsy, doctors never could give a definite diagnosis of Alzheimer's. Rather, the diagnosis progressed over time from dementia due to "possible Alzheimer's" to "probable Alzheimer's." In later years, the medical professionals did refer to her as having Alzheimer's disease, particularly after a very revealing PET scan in 2007.

2 The Early Years Of Alzheimer's

a) Early Diagnosis

I can't stress strongly enough the importance of early diagnosis. I know sometimes there's an inclination to put off getting a diagnosis, hoping to lengthen the time of denial or at least not hear the words spoken. But by getting an early diagnosis for my mother, I was able to coordinate daily living adjustments and compromises, along with medical treatment, which kept her in her own home for over four years. So I'm speaking to those with beginning symptoms of dementia as well as concerned family members: it is in everyone's best interests to get that early diagnosis to both start treatment and plan for the future. The earlier the diagnosis, the sooner medication can begin to slow the progression and the more involved in future plans the afflicted person can be if he or she so chooses.

Finding the right place to diagnose your loved one is important. The first stop was her primary care physician. My mother told her doctor she was hearing voices, so he referred her to a psychiatrist. Having had my mother explain to me that the auditory hallucinations were not audible voices, but simply an arbitrary word popping into her head on occasion, I did not think this was the most appropriate referral. So I called the psychiatrist prior to the appointment. After discussing her symptoms with him, he agreed he was not the best resource to evaluate her.   He recommended a local program called the Memory Disorders Program.   This was a nice confirmation for me since that same program had been recommended to me by other professionals in the Assisted Living and dementia care facilities I had been speaking with.

I made an appointment with the Memory Disorders Program and was impressed with it very quickly.   The program consisted of a psychiatrist, a neuropsychologist, a neurologist, and a clinical nurse specialist (RN / NP) who was the primary contact and coordinated the entire program. Mom had an initial appointment with each of the four, and then a plethora of both physical and mental tests. Everything from blood tests (to check for deficiencies that can cause dementia) to CAT scans to neurological and psychological testing.   Since the only definitive test for Alzheimer's disease was postmortem, they worked to rule out all other possible causes, thus backing into an Alzheimer's diagnosis by the process of elimination (of everything else).   At the end of the testing, the diagnosis for my mother was dementia with the probable cause of Alzheimer's disease.

Beyond the initial diagnosis, the Memory Disorders Program became a good support system and information resource for me.   I took my mother back for follow-up appointments every three months for ongoing evaluation. The three-month visits consisted primarily of the "Mini-Mental State Exam," a 30-point interactive exam that took approximately 20 minutes and was used to detect and track the progression of cognitive impairment.   Additionally, there was a short conversation with both my mother and me to discuss any changes I had been seeing since the prior visit and any concerns my mother had. Annually, the lengthy three to four hour neuropsychological exam was given to mark the progression of her dementia. This was only done twice for my mother — once upon initial evaluation and once at the one year mark. After that, my mother vehemently did not want to participate in it. So we stopped doing the exam, because it was not worth upsetting her simply to confirm through testing what I was witnessing on an ongoing basis.

At the initial testing, and for about the first two years, my mother continued to score high on the "Mini-Mental State Exam," ranging from 27 to 29 out of 30 points. This was always surprising to both the clinical nurse and me because we could see the definite progression of her dementia in several areas of her daily living. It is not uncommon for someone in this early stage of dementia to appear fine in conversations (especially to strangers who don't know if something said is false) but demonstrate notable functional problems in daily life.

b) Treatment

There are a variety of medications to treat Alzheimer's-related dementia. Once your loved one is diagnosed, your physician(s) should recommend a course of action. Do not be afraid to ask about the pros and cons of the different medications. The Memory Disorders Program prescribed Aricept for my mother, starting with a low dosage and building up to 10 mg per day over several weeks. While she did experience the side effect of nausea, she did not connect that to the new prescription, so she did not stop taking it. I brought her a nice blend of red tea that I liked. Fortunately, she liked it and felt it helped settle her stomach while she got used to the medication. Soon, even before she built up to the 10 mg dosage, the symptom of nausea went away. The addition of Aricept was the only medical treatment given. At one point I asked about adding an antidepressant (such as Zoloft), and the Memory Disorders Program concurred, but my mother refused to consider that. Zoloft was suggested due to existing depression that was not directly related to the dementia.

c) First Lifestyle Changes

At first there may be few, if any, lifestyle changes. I consider us very lucky that Mom responded so well to the Aricept. At that time (2004), we were told that, at best, Aricept would stabilize her for 6 to 12 months with minimal progression of the disease; then, it would become ineffective and she would begin to decline. However, Mom stabilized for a good 18 to 24 months before I noticed any real decline. Thereafter, the decline was slow, but constant, for the next year. During this time Mom continued to live alone, take care of herself (cooking, cleaning, laundry, etc.) and drive. As the disease progressed, I began to adapt her home and put processes in place to compensate for what she was having trouble doing.

I created a set of private web pages (which evolved over time as new needs arose) that I could access online from anywhere, so I always had her information available to me from home, work, or any place where I could access the internet on a computer. This proved invaluable, particularly when I was at work 50 miles from my mother's home. One of the first pages I created had all her utility account numbers and customer service phone numbers, so I was able to deal with a utility company (usually the telephone company) to straighten out changes to her service that often resulted from a cold sales call that had gotten her to agree to things that not only she didn't need, but also were bad for her in her current condition. I had a page with images of all her pills, so when she asked me about one during her daily 7:00 a.m. pill call I would know which pill she was talking about and I could tell her what it was for. I had a page with an image of her prescription bottle labels, so I could easily reorder the prescriptions on the 1st of each month from wherever I was and pick them up on the way to her house (it took a few months to sync them to the 1st of each month). I had a page with all her doctors' names/numbers and hospital names/numbers as well as a page with pictures of her medical insurance cards. Other information on the pages included her local repair services, police department, and senior center. One of the last pages I created was a picture of her microwave panel, so I could talk her through heating a frozen dinner. I could also bring up a copy of her *Health Care Proxy*, *Power of Attorney*, and *Letter of Activation*, which I was able to conveniently access from a hospital computer during an unexpected emergency room admission. All this allowed me to efficiently manage and compensate for the areas in which she was failing, whether I was home, at work, or elsewhere.

I happen to be an IT professional, so creating personal webpages was a natural solution for me in the technology available in 2004. Find a way that is natural for you to have this information available to you at all times. In today's world, with smartphones and tablets so commonly used, simply saving information in logical groupings that can be easily accessed might be a good solution. The goal is to ensure that you can resolve your loved one's issues as quickly as possible, with the least resistance, from wherever you are when the issue arises.

3 The Ongoing Progression

a) A Few More Changes

After the initial 18 months on Aricept, Mom's dementia slowly progressed and her ability to safely and satisfactorily tend to all her daily needs became challenging. After six months of this gradual decline, she became extremely indecisive. Even with small things, she simply was unable to make a decision. In the grocery store, she no longer could decide which items to select and place in her cart. She would sometimes stand and stare at the bread selection for 20 minutes and still not be able to choose one (even though she had always bought the same bread for years), or olive oil, or canned tomatoes — things she had always bought weekly but now could no longer choose. I suspect some of it was a fear of choosing wrong, and since she couldn't remember which items she usually chose, she wouldn't select any. She also had the same problem when I would take her clothes shopping. At one point she needed a few new basic items (underwear, pants, and shirts). I took her to at least a dozen stores over a few weeks. After exhausting her store choices, I took her to some higher-end mall stores with dedicated saleswomen who would spend an hour or more with her selecting and trying on many items, but Mom could never make a decision to buy even one thing. The groceries were not a problem for me, as I was able to easily shop with her (or for her) and make the selections. However, clothes shopping, particularly women's clothes shopping, was just not an area in which I was very helpful. I was grateful Auntie Ellie was able to provide some assistance with that.

Probably the biggest concern at this 24-month mark (after beginning Aricept) was her inability to properly take her medications. I had created a system for her with a pill case that I would fill each weekend. At first, that worked. As more confusion and uncertainty set in, I revised things by eliminating the mid-day pills, leaving only the morning and evening pills. I would call her at 7:00 a.m. from work every day and Auntie Ellie would call her every evening at 7:00 p.m. to take her pills. That worked for a while. But then it became difficult to talk her through taking the right compartment on the right day, and I was never sure until I got there on the weekend what she had taken. Fortunately, Mom was not on any life-critical medications and only two prescriptions overall, one of which was Aricept. Also fortunately, she would skip doses rather than double up, so I was lucky in that respect.

b) How Much Is Too Much?

As your loved one has difficulty with more and more daily living issues, it's often easy to identify and compensate for them one at a time without ever standing back and seeing the big picture, until something occurs to make you do that. That was the mode I was in. I was continually adjusting things to accommodate her new deficiencies as they arose, and things seemed to be going fairly smoothly. Then one day on my weekend visit I found a pan of raw meatloaf (topped with ketchup) in her refrigerator. This was not uncommon because she might put it together one day, be too tired to bake it, and would refrigerate it overnight and cook it the next day. However, there was a corner square of it missing. When questioned, she said, "Oh, I ate that for lunch." I said, "But Mom, this meatloaf is raw; it hasn't been cooked yet." Her unconcerned reply was "Well, it tasted good anyway." Apparently, after saving it overnight to cook the next day, she forgot it wasn't cooked — but more importantly, did not notice that it was raw while eating it. Eating raw hamburger with raw eggs in it was a bit much for me, so that weekend my project was to remove all food from her home that had to be cooked, and stock it with microwavable dinners. She was happy about that as she had gotten a bit leery of using the oven, and even the toaster oven. That worked for quite a while, toward the end with me talking her through, on the phone, which buttons on the microwave to push to cook a pre-packaged meal (that was when the webpage with the microwave panel came to be). As much as I knew Mom should be in an Assisted Living facility at this point, she was adamantly opposed to it: so she remained in her home.

c) When It's Gone Too Far

Eventually, I went through several levels of food changes to ensure that she had food in the house she could make and eat that was not too challenging or dangerous for her to prepare. Once the microwave dinners became too challenging and frustrating for her (even with me talking her through it on the phone), I found toaster food. Much like Pop-Tarts, but some had ham and cheese, sausage and egg, and other foods in them. The selection wasn't great, but enough that I knew she could put them in the toaster and have warm food to eat. I had always kept her house stocked with staples such as tuna, peanut butter, canned vegetables and fruit, etc., so she still had those fallbacks. Eventually though, she stopped eating much savory food and simply ate whatever sweets were in the house – I later learned that this is not uncommon among Alzheimer's patients. I had to be careful when shopping for her to no longer buy large cakes and pies as she'd eat the entire thing within a few hours and nothing else the rest of the day. I found small single or double serving pies and such for her.

There were some services covered by her insurance such as weekly light housecleaning and the Meals on Wheels program. Although I spoke with Mom on the phone at least a couple of times a day, I was only able to get to her house on weekends. So I set up the light housecleaning service for Wednesdays; that way, I knew she'd be seen by someone halfway between my visits. I also set up the daily Meals on Wheels service. However, neither of those services lasted long as my mother was not on board with them, especially when she quickly realized they were not there to socialize with her — which was her goal in allowing someone to come.

Also at this time, I was forced to disable Mom's car. The medical professionals involved told me that because I knew she shouldn't be driving, if I didn't prevent her from driving, I could be liable if she were in an accident and damaged property, or worse, human life. When my mother threatened to buy or rent a car I became concerned, especially since I was only getting to her house on weekends. The Memory Disorders Program said that they could notify the Registry of Motor Vehicles and have her license revoked, which might drive home the point to her that she could no longer drive (and also prevent her from buying or renting a car), but it would be very emotional for her. Fearing both the danger to Mom, and the potential liability to me, I advised them to go ahead and do that. This was something I later regretted, and still regret to this day. When my mother received the letter in the mail from the Registry of Motor Vehicles that her driver's license had been revoked for medical reasons, she broke down and sobbed. I hadn't seen her so deeply hurt since my oldest brother passed away decades before. I'm not sure if it was the finality of the loss of independence or if she felt she was being stripped of her dignity and was now being treated as less than an adult, but it was extremely emotional for her. In hindsight, I had become too focused on the slight possibility that her hollow threats and venting (to buy or rent a car) might become a reality. If I had known how deeply losing her license would hurt her, I would've never allowed that to happen.

By now, I knew Mom should not be living alone. I again encouraged her to move to an Assisted Living facility that we had toured, but she still refused.

4 When They Can't Live At Home Any Longer

At some point, a dementia patient will no longer be safe living on his or her own. This is always distressing to both the patient and the primary decision-maker, and the timing is never easy.

Being pragmatic by nature, I thought it would be good to have my mother be a part of the moving decision early on and have input into the choices and decisions. I surveyed and picked the best Assisted Living facility covered by her insurance and brought her there by appointment for lunch, a tour, and a discussion with the admissions staff. I thought it would be better for Mom to move there sooner, even while she was still driving (she could have her car there). Then she'd have made the decision herself and become familiar with the place, routine, and staff; that way, when she reached the point where she was unable to live alone, she'd already be there and it would not be strange to her.

Of course, that was not my mother's point of view. She enjoyed the lunches and tours and said the place was beautiful, but not for her. Her decision was that she'd stay in her home until she couldn't and then I could do what I wanted. She insisted that by the time it was necessary for her to move, she would not know anything, so she wouldn't care. Of course, that was not the case, nor did I expect it to be. I knew that her inability to safely live alone would come long before she would be unaware of her surroundings.

a) Proactive Or Emergency?

If decisions can be made early on with the patient, that would seem to be the best path. Even if the move is delayed until necessary, at least the patient would still have input into his or her future.   In an ideal situation, the patient would agree to move to a place with assistance earlier than necessary to avoid an emergency situation. That was not my mother's choice.

So I was forced to live with the emergency situation route. This was especially difficult for me as her primary caregiver and decision-maker. As she became less and less able to handle normal daily tasks and to eat properly, I became more and more stressed and worried about the inevitable emergency that would trigger the move (and then to where?). The stress was augmented by the fact that I lived 20 miles from her and worked another 30 miles in the opposite direction, putting me 50 miles away from her while at work — and thus, only getting to her house on the weekends except in an emergency.

b) The Terrible *Too's*

I named this period the Terrible *Too's* because there may come a time when your loved one is *Too Cognitive* to be forced to move against their will and yet *Too Demented* to be able to safely live on their own. My mother was *Too Cognitive* because she was able to firmly voice her desire that she not be moved from her home, and she hadn't done anything the *system* considered *Too Dangerous* to be moved against her will. Yet she was *Too Agitated, Too Afraid, Too Unable To Eat Properly, Too Unable To Take Her Medications Properly*, and *Too Demented* to safely live alone. Because I knew it was only a matter of time before she endangered herself, it was a period of intense stress and fear for me, amplified by my distance from her.

During this period she would call me at work in hysterics about someone being in her bathroom mirror. Since it was her own reflection, she often thought it was one of her sisters trapped in there and she was going to break the mirror to save her. Other times, she'd think it was a stranger who had stolen her favorite earrings and jewelry — because, of course, she could see them being worn by her reflection. Either way, she'd be hysterical, so I'd leave work and drive the 50 miles to her house. Most times, by the time I arrived she had calmed down and forgotten all about it. Out of fear that she would one day try to break the mirror and it or the broken glass would come down on her, I covered the bathroom mirror with a large piece of cardboard. Mom liked that, but then made me cut a little flap in the cardboard that she could open to see her face to put on her makeup in the mornings. Nothing was going to extinguish the "girly-girl" in her.

As Mom's dementia and hallucinations worsened, she came to believe that the people on TV were real. During the day this was positive, as they became her friends and she talked to them. At night, she would accidentally channel surf to less appropriate shows and then be afraid of the people. So for quite a stretch, every night between midnight and 2:00 a.m., either my Aunt Ellie or I would get a call from Mom. She was terrified of these people and said she was going to run out of the house to get away from them. It would take an hour to talk her down and finally get her to change the channel or shut off the TV (she was afraid they would come after her if she switched them off).

I knew it was only a matter of time before she ran out in the middle of the night, got cut from breaking a mirror, or did some other act to place herself in danger — and I was terrified.

c) Do You Have The Legal Authority?

Laws differ from state to state, and hopefully are evolving for the better; but you may find that even when it is in your loved one's best interests to be moved, you may not have the legal authority to do so. When I realized it was no longer safe for Mom to live on her own, I tried desperately to get her into an Assisted Living facility. We were several years into our once-every-three-months check-ups with the Memory Disorders Program, so I went to them first. Although they agreed she was unsafe and should not be living alone, they could not order her move, nor could I — even with the *Health Care Proxy* and *Power of Attorney* I had for her. I had her evaluated in her home by a visiting nurse practitioner who also agreed she was unsafe and should not be living alone, but concurred that neither she nor I could move Mom against her wishes. I called Adult Protective Services and explained all the reasons she was unsafe and that all medical evaluations agreed. I was asked if she had started a fire or wandered out at night, and I said, "Not yet, but it is inevitable based on what is happening". They also agreed 100% that she was unsafe at home, but she could not be moved without her consent until she endangered herself.

I finally sought out an elder law attorney in my state. He informed me that the only way to move my mother against her will was to obtain guardianship over her. He also emphatically recommended against me doing that. In addition to the high cost of the process, he said she would be appointed an attorney and I would have to prove to the judge, in front of her with her attorney defending her, that she was incompetent. He said the trauma of that and the resulting damaged relationship would be much more negative for both of us than not moving her. He believed that her need to continue to trust me throughout the rest of her life was more important than moving her against her wishes.

The gray area, or gap, in the laws that protect the rights of the elderly (and all people) versus those that protect their safety are frustrating. I had to accept that I simply had to wait until she did something the *system* recognized as placing herself in danger and hope it was caught before she was actually harmed by it. This was an extremely stressful time for me.

d) Selecting A Facility

Choosing a facility can be a daunting task but is not one to leave to chance when it's for the rest of your loved one's life. Once Mom actually put herself in danger (by wandering out in the middle of the night in sleet and freezing rain in her nightgown and slippers), she had been transported by ambulance (from where she was found) to the emergency room (ER). I left work and drove the 60 miles to the hospital, stopping at her house on the way to secure it as the police had said she left all the doors and windows open. The ER was simply going to send her back home after examining her and finding no physical injuries. I refused to take her home and insisted that the ER call in Adult Protective Services. Once Adult Protective Services became involved, they placed Mom in a nursing home (she was beyond Assisted Living at this point) on an emergency basis. The nursing home was crowded and had nothing to offer for dementia patients, but she was safe and that gave me the opportunity over the next few days, when I wasn't visiting Mom, to tour local dementia units. In my opinion, there was only one that stood out as the best, so I applied there. We were lucky it only took five weeks for an opening to occur. I finally had Mom in a safe place that was bright, pleasant, staffed with dementia trained professionals, and had activity programs for dementia patients.

Whenever possible, try to find a facility that has a unit dedicated to dementia patient care and quality of life. This is the most appropriate especially when the patient is still highly functional – although they cannot live alone, they can converse, they know their immediate caregivers, and they can participate in activities designed for their current level of dementia. Be aware that most dementia units will eventually move a patient in the later stages to a regular long-term care unit to open up a spot for a waiting highly functional dementia patient.

Nursing homes get a bad rap much of the time, and that's because we often only hear about the negative experiences. I have found that overall, nursing home employees are wonderful people and caregivers and are there because they care. While, as in any profession, you may get the occasional bad staff member, they normally don't last long. The real shortcomings of nursing homes are insufficient budgets and short-staffed shifts that are as frustrating for the staff as for the patients and family members.

e) Helping Your Loved One Settle In

While transitioning a loved one into a facility is never easy for either the patient or the caregiver, some things can ease your loved one's adjustment to the new facility, such as: having a more *acceptable reason* for their going there and keeping everyone on the same page with that reason, and having some of their personal belongings decorating their new space when they arrive. For my *acceptable reason* for her being in the first nursing home, I used her complaint that her legs hurt her and said she was there to have them looked at by the doctor. When the move to the second nursing home came, I told her that the place she was in was more of a hospital, and the good news is the doctor said she didn't need to be there any longer – but that he also said she wasn't ready to go home alone yet either, so she was being transferred to another place to help her get her strength back.

Although the first nursing home my mother was admitted to on an emergency basis was completely inappropriate for her condition, she was resistant to leaving. She was in an old institutional-looking room with very old furnishings and four patient beds, and she was not able to communicate with any of the three patients in her room. Because it was not a lockdown unit, she had to wear an electronic device that would not allow her to use elevators or enter stairwells and would beep loudly if she attempted to leave the L-shaped unit. Unless I was there at mealtime to take her, she was not able to eat in the dining room as it was not in her unit and there was no available staff to accompany her. She was not allowed to participate in any activities, again because they were not on her unit. During the five weeks she was at this facility, as often as possible I went when there was an activity I knew she'd enjoy and I took her to it. As bad of an environment as this was for her condition, she became accustomed to it and did not wish to leave. Part of this was due to her increased resistance to change, but a large part was due to the wonderful staff she came to know.

After five weeks in the first nursing home, I got the call that there was an opening in the dementia unit I had applied for at another nursing home. To make it as easy a transition as possible, I went there first and decorated her new room with things from her house so she would be surrounded by her familiar belongings, many of which were her own artwork. Once that was accomplished, I went to the first nursing home and packed up her belongings. Mom was giving me the cold shoulder because she did not want to leave. Unfortunately, with three shifts of staff, the agreed-upon reason given to Mom for the change of facility was not adhered to; so, I became the culprit. I had prearranged a transport van for Mom as I did not want to be in a problematic situation during transport if she began insisting on going home. I had also asked that she be given an Ativan (an anti-anxiety medication) 30 minutes before the transport time, so it would be a calm process for her rather than an agitated one.

Once her belongings were packed into my car, I waited with her for the transport van, walked with her to the van where I told her I'd see her in a few minutes, and then I raced to the new facility so I would be standing there waiting when the van arrived. I did not want her to feel alone or abandoned in the process. Auntie Ellie also met me there so we were both there to greet Mom when she was wheeled out of the van.

The new unit was bright and cheery with only two beds per room, more closet space, nicer furniture, and more drawer space. I had already decorated the walls with all her personal belongings from home, which she immediately recognized and happily said, "Here's all my stuff; I wondered what had happened to it." The unit manager and I got Mom acclimated to the new unit and staff. When it was time for lunch, Mom had a place set for her with her name on a fancy name card in front of her plate. Finally, Mom looked at me and said, "I know you said this place would be nicer, but I didn't realize it would be this beautiful." Mom had not only forgiven me for moving her, but was thankful. More importantly, being a dementia unit that was closely following the definition for a *Homestead Unit*, Mom was now in a place that could meet her needs, offer activities at her level, and help me to give her the best quality of life she could achieve.

f) Augmenting Facility Care

Once your loved one is a resident of a facility, your involvement in their care should not end. Understandably, relationships are different, distances are different, and personal schedules allow for different levels of involvement. My point here is that while your loved one is now safe from wandering or harming themselves, they still need as much involvement as you can give them to ensure they receive both the best care possible at that facility and that they are continually living the best quality of life possible throughout the rest of their lives.

I was extremely fortunate that this *Homestead Unit* was headed by a very involved non-medical unit manager who was easy to deal with and was very interested in ensuring that my mother was living up to her quality of life potential. Consequently, she not only allowed and assisted in implementing many of my suggestions but where they made sense she used us as a pilot program which, once proven successful, she was able to offer to other residents.

One of the first things I suggested was that my mother get involved in as many activities that her level of cognition would allow, many of which were not in the dementia unit. The dementia unit cycled over time, with the bulk of the population going from mostly highly functional to mostly end stage. At the time my mother arrived, the activities were more geared toward less functional, later stage dementia patients. She was always included, but there were higher-level activities throughout the other long term care units in the facility that she was also capable of participating in and were more appropriate for her at her level of functionality. So, with their permission, each month I would get the monthly activities calendar for the entire building. I'd circle the activities I felt my mother would enjoy (bingo, bowling, etc.) and give it back to the unit manager. My mother could be walked to the other unit for these activities and left unattended by her unit staff, as the activity was run by staff from the other unit. I had been concerned that the other unit staff running the activities would resent my mother joining their activity — as, at the very least, it was yet one more person for them to watch and interact with. To my surprise, the other unit staff was so happy to have more participants that they welcomed my mother and treated her as one of their own residents. More often than not, they didn't even call back down to Mom's dementia unit at the activity's end for one of her aides to come and get her, but would simply walk her down themselves.

Unfortunately, we quickly learned that simply returning the monthly activity calendar with my chosen activities circled was ineffective. Regular staff simply didn't have the time to monitor this brand new additional task for one resident and never remembered to check it.   So, my involvement with her activities then became daily. I kept the monthly activity calendar with me. From work, I would call her unit nurses' station about 20 to 30 minutes before the start of each activity I wanted her to attend. That gave them time to make sure she was freshened up and to coordinate someone to walk her over. It worked great: her staff was happy to not have to remember to check the calendar and Mom got to all these extra activities she would have not participated in otherwise. Yes, it meant that once or twice a day I called from work to ask them to take her; but I was happy to do it and always felt content afterwards knowing she was enjoying herself rather than sitting and watching TV or doing an activity that was not challenging to her. It also had the extra advantage of my mother feeling that she was "going out" to bingo, which was very reminiscent of when she lived at home and would do so, as well as not making her feel "locked in" to a unit she could never leave. Soon after this began to run smoothly, her unit manager started sending other appropriate residents to these activities with her.

g) Managing Medications in the Facility

Keeping yourself in the loop with your loved one's medications once they are in a nursing home may be something you have to continually address. Throughout Mom's nine years in the nursing homes (both the first short-term facility and the second permanent facility) this became a frustrating struggle that I never could solve, but had to settle for keeping on top of.

Because of my instructions as Mom's *Health Care Proxy*, as well as state and federal laws regulating specific medications (such as an antipsychotic), they were not supposed to give Mom any medication without my approval. However that almost never happened no matter how many times I called them out on it. This was probably the only issue that I became very confrontational about. Fortunately, since I visited Mom most days, and most of those visits were during either a morning or evening pill dispensing, I stayed on top of any changes they slipped in without my knowledge or approval. When confronted, they would agree that they could not give my mother anything without my approval — even while I was telling them they just had. Talk about frustrating!

The first violation occurred in her first week in the first nursing home. Due to Mom's hallucinations, they put her on Seroquel (an antipsychotic). After *Googling* this drug and finding it had a black box warning specifically for elderly dementia patients, I naturally was very opposed to it and immediately stopped it. However, nursing home doctors often know best, even when writing prescriptions against warnings. I was assured that in spite of the black box warning on the drug, it was used all the time in cases like my mother's. Given Mom's agitated, fearful state much of the time, as well as her occasional aggressive state, and after checking with other medical professionals (including the *Memory Disorders Program*) who agreed with the use of Seroquel, I did submit to a trial. For us, the results were miraculous. Her hallucinations stopped immediately as well as all the fears and torment that accompanied them. I decided to focus on her daily comfort and contentment and not worry about long term issues. Her daily terrors and anguish were gone, she was content, and I would deal with issues that may arise five or ten years down the road at that time.

But I still needed to stay involved as the Seroquel made her too drowsy all day long and they didn't appear to be concerned about that. So, I worked with them to decrease and eventually eliminate the morning dose and reduce the bedtime dose. Soon we had the correct dosage for Mom, taken only at bedtime. She slept well because of taking it at bedtime (so all her night terrors stopped) and while it stayed in her system enough throughout the next day to continue to prevent the hallucinations, it was no longer at a level that made her drowsy, so she could participate in activities and eat all her meals normally. If I hadn't persisted and stayed involved I'm not sure if, or how quickly, these adjustments would have been made.

Another time (much later in the second nursing home) I found they were suddenly giving Mom cholesterol medications. I was livid, as my mother had tried those long before the Alzheimer's and they gave her such severe leg cramps she chose to stop taking them. I knew she didn't want to be on them. As her advocate, it was my responsibility to consider her wishes when deciding on treatment and care plans. I also saw no benefit to treating such things (especially against her wishes) now that she had a terminal illness. I stopped them immediately and once again, reminded them of their legal obligation to inform me and get my approval before giving her any new medications.

These are just two examples, of many, where the nursing home doctor or nurse practitioner overstepped their boundaries and prescribed new medications without first getting my approval, or even informing me. Fortunately, I was there so often I always discovered it within a day or two. But no matter how many times this occurred, keeping me in the loop was simply not something they could seem to do regularly (although there were instances when they did comply with the approval process). I do not believe there was any malice or ill intent in bypassing me — it simply seemed to be too inconvenient and outside of their process.

5 Interacting With Your Loved One As The Alzheimer's Progresses

The basic theme of this section is adapting to your loved one's needs on an ongoing basis. Things change from day to day and week to week. What worked yesterday may not work tomorrow. Often they will let you know when it is time for the change; other times, you will have to decide a change is needed based on ineffectively trying to accomplish something that no longer works. Many of these adaptations can be very simple, straight forward, and inexpensive; yet, they are not always in the nursing home's bag of tricks nor did I always think of them right away.

a) Redefining Your Relationship

Probably the most consistent thing throughout Mom's 13-year struggle with Alzheimer's was that no accommodation I put into place for her lasted very long. It was a continuous reevaluation of her needs and what would help accommodate each need, both while she was living in her home and later in the nursing home. I often say that I lost my father once, when he died, but I lost my mother over and over and over again each time her dementia worsened and reduced her abilities to another level. Each time, in addition to losing more functionality and cognition, she would lose a little more of herself. Each time she was a slightly different person that I had to once again get to know, understand, learn to communicate with, and learn how to make her the most comfortable and content. My goal was to always give her the best quality of life she was capable of achieving at whatever level she was at in any given moment.

b) Recreating Activities

During the time Mom was in the *Homestead Unit,* there was the wonderful advantage that they engaged her throughout the day with activities suited for her level of cognition and functionality (in addition to the off-unit activities I had her sent to during her highly functional period). So beyond coordinating her involvement in the off-unit activities to augment her day, I was not too concerned with her facility activities (this would later change when she was transferred out of the dementia unit). Throughout her highly functional years I would take her out at least once a week on my own. We'd go to lunch and a store of her choice, or on a picnic by a pond where we could feed the ducks, or to the local zoo.

Once Mom could no longer go to the toilet by herself, I was no longer able to take her out for very long alone or she'd soil herself. So our excursions went from half days to an hour or less. I found a take-out ice cream stand that also served hot dogs, hamburgers, etc., and it was only a few miles from the nursing home. They had some minimal outdoor seating which we used. While a much scaled-down version of our prior outings, we could get there, Mom could eat her foot-long hot dog, curly fries, and soda and we could be back to the nursing home in an hour — just in time for her to get assistance using the bathroom.

As Mom's motor skills declined and she needed a wheelchair for all but a few short steps, I obtained a light-weight wheelchair that I could fold up and take with us. As time went on and Mom declined more, I could no longer get her into and out of the car by myself. My first inclination was to think our days of going out were over, but I felt it was so important for her to leave the facility periodically, both for a change of scenery and to have different experiences. I hired a private CNA (Certified Nurse's Aide) to accompany us. This was an added expense, so our excursions went from once a week to twice a month. But having the private CNA with us increased our outings back up to half-day excursions since the CNA could assist her in the restroom wherever we were.

Once a month we would go to Mom's sister's for lunch. When we were able to embark on a second monthly outing, we'd often have lunch at a mall restaurant. After lunch, Mom could window shop some of the stores from her wheelchair, although she primarily enjoyed just sitting in the center of the mall to people watch. She especially enjoyed seeing children as they passed by. As Mom's decline continued, suddenly the restaurant and mall she had enjoyed so much for many months became overwhelming for her. As her world became smaller, the activity level around her became too much and she went from enjoying the experience to becoming anxious and agitated and asking to leave. So I stopped the public outings and reduced our excursions to the once-a-month lunches at my Aunt Ellie's, where Mom was comfortable because it was just her sister and brother-in-law as well as the three of us (the CNA, Mom and me). Eventually, Mom became completely wheelchair-bound, and was placed into and removed from the wheelchair with a lift. I adjusted once again and engaged a wheelchair van for the monthly lunch trips to Auntie Ellie's. Those monthly lunches continued until my aunt became ill and could no longer host them — about 19 months before Mom passed.

Once my mother was wheelchair-bound and transferred into the non-dementia long term care unit, she had more of a need for supplemental activities. As we were down to only the once-a-month outings, I made it a point to take her outside whenever the weather permitted. The nursing home she was in was one of four on a large campus; additionally, there was an Assisted Living facility on campus. Sometimes we'd sit under the covered front of her building, or spend time in the courtyard, or use the second-floor covered porch. Depending on the weather and her mood I might wheel her across the street where behind another building was a small fish pond. A couple of times each summer the Assisted Living facility would host outdoor concerts with local talent and I would wheel Mom the quarter of a mile to those. As with the mall, Mom went from enjoying the outdoor concerts to becoming overwhelmed and agitated, so I stopped bringing her to them.

A few years later, on a whim, I ended up taking her to the last outdoor concert of that summer because our evening had just played out perfectly (Mom finished dinner early, she stayed awake, she was content, the weather was perfect, and we had gone outside at the right time to head down to the concert). The concert genres were all different, but in keeping with our perfect evening, this one happened to be Mom's all-time favorite music: '50's and '60's country songs. We stayed way back this time so she was not overwhelmed by the crowd and the music was not too loud for her. When we got back to our building and were in the elevator, I nonchalantly said, "I enjoyed that; I hope you enjoyed it too." At that time Mom rarely talked, and even more rarely, made sense if she did, so I was not expecting a response. But Mom looked up at me with filled eyes, and with every ounce of control she could muster, she struggled to verbalize the most heartfelt "Thank you," as if I had given her the world, or a meal when she hadn't eaten for a month.

It made me choke up to realize how bored she must have been, and I suddenly felt that I had failed her. Rather than stopping the concerts altogether when she became agitated at them, I wished I had thought of trying the compromise to attend them from a distance, as we had done that day. That's when I decided I had to figure out something more to do for her ongoing entertainment. I began creating half-hour video concerts (from YouTube downloads) of her favorite country songs, Italian songs, Christmas songs, etc. For the last two years of Mom's life, once or twice a week (depending on her alertness), I'd wheel her down to the rarely used private living room/library and hook up my USB interface to the large, wall-mounted flat-screen TV. She'd watch and enjoy her private concerts while holding my two fingers (as she always did).

Other times we'd sit in the lobby, sometimes watching the TV there, sometimes playing solitaire on the computer, and sometimes just visiting — but primarily, getting her off her unit for a change of scenery.

I learned to view meals as an activity. It doesn't take much time spent in a nursing home to realize that mealtime is a major event that is looked forward to by the residents. I always tried to make it more than just a meal by having one of Mom's favorite music CDs playing quietly next to us, putting a rose or other decoration on the table, or setting our table away from the crowd — sometimes outside on the balcony in the nice weather for our own private picnic.

I also got permission to take Mom to breakfast in the common dining room. Only those who could order food, feed themselves, and had no choking issues were allowed to eat in that dining room, so the majority of residents ate in their own units, assisted by staff. But because I was with Mom, they allowed me to take her. The tables were set up in restaurant fashion and there was a short-order cook at the front. You could order eggs (cooked any way), pancakes, waffles, etc. along with breakfast meats and potatoes, all cooked to order. So for Mom, it was "going out to eat." Even once she declined to the level of being restricted to pureed foods (due to swallowing/choking issues) and I made and pureed her food at home, I would still bring her there with my homemade pureed breakfast foods and feed her there, in our little restaurant.

c) White Lies

One area that caused me great conflict was the need to lie to my mother. I'm not one who lies by nature or habit and always believed in being honest with Mom, even upon the development of her dementia. I quickly learned that there was a time to tell white lies for her sake, to not create a confrontation or cause her undue stress or grief.

The easy lies were the harmless ones, the ones that didn't matter or evoke any emotion (and in fact kept her content). For instance, rather than correcting my mother I realized it was far more compassionate to make up little white lies to appease her.

When I'd mention something that I knew I had told her already, and she'd accuse me of never having told her that, I'd say, "I'm sorry Mom, I thought I told you, but sometimes I forget things." This gave a two-fold benefit. First, because it was said sincerely and apologetically (as if it were true), it put all the fault on me, and my mother's response was to immediately forgive me. Second, it validated for her that it was okay to forget things; it was not something to hide, defend, or be embarrassed about. This comforted her because she knew she was forgetting things.

The tricky lies (which I never mastered) were the ones where great emotion was involved. And my mother was coy, and would sometimes test my aunt and me with things she knew. If we lied to save her grief, she would call us out on it. If we didn't lie, and she wasn't testing us, then she'd naturally become upset over the topic. One great source of anxiety for all of us was when she had more or less forgotten that family members, such as her parents, had died many years before. She would ask about her mother, for instance. Unfortunately, her loss of these memories was not linear. One day she'd remember, another she wouldn't, then she'd flip back again — so we were always on guard and never knew how to answer. If she had truly forgotten at that moment, and we said that her mother had passed long ago, she'd get upset as if she were just learning it. More poignantly, she'd be angry at us for not having told her about it all these years. On the other hand, if she did remember (or kind of remember) and we said her mother was home cooking, she'd call us out and say her mother was dead and why were we lying to her. I'm not sure whether it was more distressing for her or us. I have no real suggestions for dealing with this, other than do your best to read the situation and respond accordingly. The best advice I can give you is that if you are trying your best, accept that this happens and do not lay guilt on yourself when you respond incorrectly: sometimes, it's simply a no-win situation.

d) Dolls, Flex Straws, And Mittens

I like to use these three examples to convey how, as our loved one progresses through the stages of Alzheimer's, they have wants and needs that we may either resist or not immediately consider. It all comes down to adapting to the moment, and often with very simple adjustments that we may overlook.

DOLLS: When I first had my mother transferred to the permanent Alzheimer's unit I had selected, following her emergency placement in the temporary facility, I immediately noticed many residents holding dolls. At first, I was uncomfortable with the idea that my mother might one day do that too, and I did not want to encourage that. At that time, my mother was still highly functional, knew they were dolls, and had no desire to hold one. I knew the day might come when she would want one and I dreaded that day. I didn't think I would like seeing my mother cuddling a doll as if it were a real baby because that would signify that her Alzheimer's had progressed further; more so, I felt that would be demeaning for the intelligent woman I knew as my mother. However, when that time came, my experience was just the opposite. I saw the peace and comfort that holding a doll brought her, and it made me feel good to know she was content and felt secure at that moment, especially when I was leaving for the day.

And the time came sooner than I expected. We were in a dollar store during one of our weekly Friday excursions and as I went to the register she trailed behind. I was in the checkout line and realized she had gone off and I had lost sight of her. A few minutes later as I was about to leave the line to look for her, she emerged with this very small Barbie-sized doll, came up to me and in the most innocent, child-like plea asked if she could have it.

I was flooded with a mix of emotions. First, the realization that we had reached that time already; second, that I wanted her to have something better than one dollar would buy at the dollar store; third, that her plea implied she thought I might say no, which hurt me that she felt that; and lastly, her child-like innocence in the request. I said of course she could have it and told her she could have anything she wanted, and asked if she wanted to go to another store and get a bigger one. She said no, she wanted that one, so of course, I bought it for her. During the entire ride back to the nursing home she hugged and talked to it. It was small, but she had chosen it, and it brought her joy. She kept saying she had picked it off a tree and rescued it. Always wanting to better understand her, I later went back to the store to see if the dolls were on a vertical display that was perhaps tree-like in appearance, but they were just in a bin on a bottom shelf. It was quite some time before I realized the name of the store was "Dollar Tree" and she must have seen that name. I soon bought her a larger, life-like doll that she fell in love with and drew comfort from for the rest of her life.

In her later stages of dementia, when the doll became more real to her, I would get upset if I found her sitting without her doll to hold. It brought her great comfort to hold a "baby" and talk to it. In later stages, she sometimes didn't seem to know what she was holding — but at that stage, like an infant often does, her hands would want to hold something, anything, for security. If she had nothing in her hands, she'd ball up her shirt and hold that. Often I'd find her sitting with her doll, holding it by one leg, upside down, just to be gripping something. I'd ask if she held me like that when I was a baby because it would explain a few things. I found it was amazing how something I thought I would dislike (seeing my mother holding a doll) became as much a comfort to me as it was to her because when she was holding it, I knew she was content. It was especially comforting to me when she would talk to it as if it were a real baby because at that moment, she was content and felt useful while invoking the still present, basic mothering instincts. And that was all that mattered, that she was comfortable and content, whatever method that took.

During my visits I'd set the doll aside and Mom would hold my two fingers throughout the visit. But before leaving, I always made sure she had her doll and was seated in the TV/activity room.

FLEX STRAWS: As Mom progressed and her motor skills began to be affected, drinking from a glass or cup became very accident-prone. In addition to causing a clean-up incident, clothing stains, and losing the drink, it also frustrated and sometimes angered her as she'd try to find an excuse for the accident. Staff members would often put a straw in the glass, but having a straight straw unsecured in a glass just caused an additional motor skill challenge, as it either required two hands (one for the glass and one for the straw) or a very coordinated single hand approach. I purchased child straw cups at a local grocery store. They came in four-packs of assorted colors and were inexpensive. They were very basic 10-ounce plastic cups with a snap-on top that had a hole for a straw. While they came with a stiff, straight, reusable straw, I found that disposable flex straws worked best, both for my convenience of tossing them in the trash afterwards and for her positioning the cup. She did very well with these cups and flex straws, and while she always drank well, it increased her fluid intake as nobody had to sit with her and help. She could hold the cup with only one hand (since the straw was securely in place and did not move around), move the cup to put the straw to her mouth, and drink when she wanted. If she tipped or even dropped it, little or no liquid came out.

I also felt that using these at every visit reinforced the sucking action for drinking through a straw. In the later stages of Mom's illness, and at times when she was sick and not eating, simply putting a straw to her lips would invoke the drinking reflex and I was able to get nutrition into her through liquids. The nursing home did not stock flex-straws, so I always kept a package in her room.

MITTENS: After the time had passed that I could take Mom out alone, and I hired a private CNA to assist me in taking her out, I began to run into other logistical issues. Mom had some very nice gloves that she loved, so, come winter, putting them on her in preparation for an excursion became part of the ritualistic assembling of her outer winter garments. I often got teased by staff that I was overdressing her (sweater, winter coat, scarf, kerchief, and gloves) to go the few feet outside to the car and again not very far from the car to the inside of wherever our destination was. I would say it was payback for all those times when I was a small child and she dressed me so thick I could barely move or bend my knees and elbows when she'd send me out to play in the snow, and I'd very stiffly march outside thinking if I ever fell I'd never be able to get up. As Mom's dementia progressed, it became more and more difficult to get her gloves on her. She didn't understand how to do it, how to help, or even how not to impede the process. In addition to not assisting us, she unknowingly fought our attempts to get each finger and thumb into the proper finger compartments. As we'd be sliding on the glove, she would automatically close her hand to grasp whatever it was she felt was being put into her hand. After many occasions of wrestling the gloves onto her and often settling for two or three out of four fingers properly placed, the private CNA suggested that I just buy her some mittens. So simple, yet I had never thought of it. Did they even make adult mittens? My next mission: to find women's mittens. I found a nice pair and the first time we tried them out it was smooth sailing — making it easier and faster for us, and less frustrating for Mom. They slid right on, and by the time she had the reflex to clench in order to grasp what she felt against the palm of her hand, it was completely on as we only had the thumb to guide into a separate compartment. The mittens were a success and had the added bonus of keeping her always-cold hands much warmer than the gloves had.

e) They Often Understand More Than They Can Express

One theme I learned throughout the progression of Mom's dementia (unfortunately often after the fact) is that she understood much more than appearances suggested. Because she spoke less and less, and when she did she didn't always use the right words or spoke in gibberish, it seemed like she didn't necessarily understand but was simply responding to a voice with a voice. However, there were so many times that proved to be incorrect. I realized she spoke much less due to her frustration of knowing she was not able to express her thoughts. She understood most of what I said to her, and in many cases knew what she wanted to say in response, but simply could not retrieve the right words in the correct order and verbalize them. I made mistakes. There were times I automatically spoke down to her, not in a demeaning way (at least not intentionally) but as if I were speaking to a small child. I always found she responded much better when I spoke to her in a normal adult way. So I would caution you to watch out for the natural inclination to speak to a dementia patient as if addressing a child. That doesn't mean that sentences can't be simple rather than complex, and ideas can't be delivered slowly and one at a time so there's a better chance of them absorbing the thought.

Also, be careful not to discuss the patient with staff or others in front of the patient as if the patient weren't there. My mother did understand and resented being excluded, although even the staff automatically did that with me. If the topic was something I didn't want my mother to hear, I'd stop the conversation and pick it up later outside of her presence. If it was something I thought was appropriate for her to hear, I'd include my mother in the conversation by looking at her when speaking to the other person, motioning to her and/or touching her as I spoke of her, and occasionally saying "Right?" or "how does that sound to you?" — even though I didn't necessarily expect a response. Most times there would be no verbal response, but eye or facial acknowledgment that she at least understood the conversation pertained to her. And always to keep us on our toes, every so often she'd spit out an unexpected, perfectly appropriate and often humorous response, especially if her opinion differed from ours.

f) And Sometimes They Don't

While I suggest always assuming your loved one is understanding you at some level, there are times when you think they are, but it is just lost on them.

As an example, when my mother first entered the Alzheimer's unit, she was still highly functional and knew my name and knew that I was her son. I decided that by reminding her of that on a daily basis, I would be able to force that relationship memory to be retained – Alzheimer's was not going to rob us of this too! So addressing her in a familiar, fun way we had, every day at some point in our visit I would say to her, "Who's my little Mommy?" and she'd say, "Me, I am!" This went on for many months and I was certain it would keep reinforcing that relationship memory. However, one day when we engaged in our little banter, after saying, "Me, I am!" she followed up with, "How come I always have to be the little Mommy?" At some point over that span of months, she had lost the meaning of the words and it had just become a daily game to her.

g) No Credit, Just Love

A phrase that I often found myself repeating throughout her nine years at the nursing home was "It's a good thing I don't do this for credit." So often, Mom would immediately forget something I had just done for her, or more hurtful, give someone else credit for it. But I quickly found the reward was in knowing I had done my best for my mother, and not that she knew it.

One example that comes to mind is six months after she entered the Alzheimer's unit, Mom's 80th birthday was upon us. At that time Mom was still highly functional and conversant (albeit not always in reality or even on topic), and I wanted to give her the opportunity to see people she'd likely still remember (with some help) before she lost that recognition. So I threw her an 80th birthday party and invited close family (about 12 people). It was quite an undertaking at the nursing home, but I negotiated the use of their large conference/training room. I arrived an hour and a half early with the cake, ice cream, soda, and had the pizza delivery preordered for the correct time. I spent an hour rearranging the training room furniture to accommodate a head table and guests and decorated with balloons and streamers and table coverings. Although I had stopped to visit Mom for a few minutes before decorating, I did not tell her of the surprise party. Once all the guests arrived I went back to Mom's unit and escorted her to the party. It took a little explaining but she eventually understood it was her birthday party. I took many photos that I knew would be the last ones with most of those people.   The party was a nice success.

When the party was over, I escorted Mom back to her unit, then returned to spend another hour cleaning up, removing the decorations, and returning the furniture to the way I had found it. Once that was complete, I went back to the unit to visit with my mother for a little bit, as we had not had our usual one-on-one visit that day. To my delight, she had remembered the party that had ended more than an hour before.   To my dismay, she did not remember I had been present, let alone single-handedly orchestrated and executed the party, as she welcomed my visit with, "Hi honey, you just missed it; we had a big party and everyone was here." I believe that was the first time I uttered, "It's a good thing I don't do this for credit." After a moment of hurt, I also realized it didn't matter. She had had a good time, good enough that she remembered it an hour later as an event to be talked about, and seeing her happy response was enough of a reward for me.

Be reassured though, that while your loved one may not remember the individual things you do, or have an overall concept of how much you are doing, your continued presence will help keep you in their recognition.

Throughout the nine years from entering the nursing home until her passing, my mother knew me. Oh, she didn't always know my name and had long since lost the understanding that I was her son, but she knew I belonged to her — and more importantly, whenever I was with her she knew she was safe and so she was content.

Once I was in the rare situation where I was a few hours away and had gotten a call that my mother had a spell of some sort. They had put her to bed and ordered some tests, and I said while I would be on my way in minutes, it would be a few hours before I would arrive. When I walked into Mom's room there was a CNA on each side of her bed, one holding a cold washcloth on her forehead and the other taking her vitals. Both were her regular aides who she knew well, but I could see in her face how anxious and afraid she was. As I walked in I said, "Hi Mom, I'm here." Calmness immediately came to her face and her vitals normalized. One of her aides said, "She didn't even see you yet, but the second she heard your voice she completely relaxed and calmed down." Mom didn't know what was going on, why there was all this fuss about her, or why she wasn't feeling well, but as soon as she heard my voice, she knew that somehow it would all be okay now. What greater gift can we give a declining loved one than peace, comfort, and security, especially when they don't have the cognition to understand what is happening to them? And what greater reward can we receive than to know our mere presence can have such a positive effect on them?

h) Love And Enjoy Them As They Are

Learn to love and enjoy your loved one as he or she is at every moment throughout the progression of dementia. I always found things to appreciate at each stage. I enjoyed the cute, child-like innocence Mom expressed in the early stages. I laughed at many of her remarks, observations, and incorrect conclusions because, within her dementia, her logic was impeccable. I loved how she always grasped and held my two fingers throughout our visits in the later stages.

That doesn't mean after enjoying your visits there won't be tears to follow. There were times as I was driving home I would be laughing as I replayed in my head something Mom had said or done during our visit — then, I would suddenly begin crying at the realization of how much of who she had been was lost.

The point is to focus on positives when you're together, so the visits are enjoyable for both of you. Avoid the natural inclination to correct or try to teach your loved one as you would a child. Remember, Alzheimer's patients are regressing back to a child-like understanding, but unlike a child at the same level of understanding, they are not able to progress forward.

6 Medical and Legal Issues

a) Health Care Proxy, Power of Attorney, And Activation

I am so thankful that I had the foresight, and my mother was on board with getting a *Health Care Proxy* (HCP) and *Power of Attorney* (POA) in order. We did this about nine months prior to making the appointment for her memory symptoms in the 2002-2003 timeframe. While she was starting to display some forgetfulness, this preceded, and was not prompted by, the Alzheimer's diagnosis. It was simply prudent life planning as she aged. The time to do these things is when you are healthy. But certainly, at the onset of symptoms, or a diagnosis, if you don't have these documents already in place, get them in place immediately. Since she was my *Health Care Proxy*, it was easy for me to approach her on the topic by suggesting we do them all together, as I was redoing my HCP, POA, and will at that time.

I found this could be done very inexpensively. While I'm not giving legal advice here, I will share my experience. By finding both *Health Care Proxy* and *Power of Attorney* forms for my state online, I was able to draw up my own documents at no cost. There are many reputable, free (or inexpensive) online offerings in these areas. I started with the official government site for my state. I took the best parts from the state forms, other online forms, and online recommendations and drew up my own documents. While not required by law in my state, I had our signatures notarized, just to add credibility. Most banks will notarize without charge as a courtesy for its customers, but even if you go to an independent notary, it's only a few dollars per document.

Again, I'm not giving legal advice here, but in my state, it was very important that the *Power of Attorney* contained the words "General" and "Durable" in it (i.e., "General Durable Power of Attorney"). This was looked for a lot when I would use it. I also added a clause in my own words to state that any itemization of powers listed in the POA was not meant to be exhaustive or limit the general powers given by the POA. I was pleased that when needed, I was able to use that POA, without question, for everything from utility changes, to life insurance surrender, to banking and real estate transactions.

The *Health Care Proxy* was important for making medical decisions for Mom without going through whatever process would have been necessary without having an HCP.

Once Mom was admitted to the nursing home, I asked for a letter of activation for both the POA and HCP, which they were happy to provide me with. Although it might not be needed, based upon the wording in both your POA and HCP, it does substantiate your right to use the documents. For me, it removed any possibility of being challenged as to whether my mother was able to make her own decisions. Knowing I had it with me always made me feel less stressed when using the POA and HCP, even though most times it wasn't needed.

If you are comfortable creating these documents on your own, it will save the fee for a lawyer to do so. If you are not comfortable doing this on your own, it is better to pay the attorney's fees than to not have these documents. An intermediate option may be to check with a legal clinic, or with a local law school that may offer the names of final year law students who may provide such services for a stipend.

I'll end this topic imploring people to have in place an HCP and POA.

For the primary caregiver, these documents are essential to perform many tasks and transactions for your loved one. It would have been impossible for me to change or end services to her phone, electricity, and cable TV without the POA. For whatever reason, the utility companies were the most inflexible and adamantly required the POA before even speaking to me about my mother's accounts. It was also the utility companies that I had to deal with the earliest in my mom's dementia progression, while she was still living at home, so it was invaluable that I had the POA and could fax it to them while dealing with a situation over the phone from work.

For the person afflicted with dementia, or for that matter, anyone in their golden years knowing eventually someone may need to make decisions for you, it is so inconsiderate not to have these documents in place. First, it gives you the ability to ensure that the person of your choice is going to make these decisions. Second, it will ease the burden on your loved one as he or she handles your affairs and makes your decisions. Your loved one will be going through a great deal of stress and emotion just having to do these tasks while dealing with the emotion of seeing you declining. Please do not add another layer of stress (and often expense) by forcing a process of getting legal authorization during a time of stress and emergency.

b) Social Security Representative Payee

This designation is solely for the purpose of managing the patient's Social Security benefits (if applicable) and unfortunately, the existence of an HCP and POA have absolutely no effect on obtaining this designation. I thought they might serve to at least clarify to the Social Security Administration (SSA) that it was my mother's intent that I handle all her affairs, because having both the HCP and POA covered all bases for both medical and financial decisions. However, the SSA has its own forms and procedure and as with most bureaucracies, no amount of common sense will make a difference. Since I already had POA, it wasn't imperative that I went through this process immediately, as the POA enabled me to sign my mother's personal checks to pay the nursing home her portion each month and spend the tiny remainder on some of her needs.

However, once I sold her residence (about 14 months after she went to the nursing home) I knew the change of address now made it necessary to obtain the designation of Representative Payee. In preparation, I had downloaded the SSA forms and had them filled out by the appropriate nursing home medical staff — but, it was a few months from the signing of the forms to my heading down to the SSA office for my afternoon of waiting. I have heard both good and bad experiences, mine was the latter. I happened to get the wrong woman, on the wrong day, and it became a long and adversarial process.

The big complaint was that the one form had been signed a few months prior, and perhaps my mother was now better. The fact that the forms stated my mother had permanent and terminal dementia due to Alzheimer's disease did not dissuade her. The fact that it was only their form that had been filled out earlier (by the original nursing home) and that I had very current other documents (like the letter of activation by the current nursing home) meant nothing. As my headache grew larger and my head pounded to where it felt like it would explode, I reached my tolerance limit. The look on my face must have shown my patience had ended, because as she took one look at me and with no further petitioning by me, she said, "OK, I'll do it."

That, of course, also showed she could have done it that easily all along with no debate or hassle: sometimes it's simply people enjoying exercising the power they have and sometimes we simply have to make the best of it. I graciously accepted her acceptance of the documents and thanked her. I was surprised by this very difficult experience as a close friend of mine had an extremely quick and easy experience with this same process when her mother had gone to a nursing home for her final days.

There was some additional follow-up, primarily with my mother's bank, to get her personal checking account changed to a Representative Payee account and have new checks printed. In contrast, this was an easy and pleasant task as the bank's personnel were compassionate and eager to help. I was able to continue using the existing checks (due to the POA) until the new checks arrived.

c) DNRs And Advanced Directives (*Making The Tough Decisions*)

DNR: Some of the most difficult decisions you'll have to make about health care are the medical treatments you will (and will not) allow for your loved one. These may change as time goes on and will likely evolve with the progression of their dementia. You do not have to make every decision immediately upon admitting your loved one to a facility. Never assume that because a choice is difficult, that it is wrong, or, because one is easy, that it is right. For me, most times, the right choice for Mom was often the most difficult to make.

When my mother was first admitted to the dementia unit, the social worker added the Advanced Directives form to the already large folder of information and paperwork I had to fill out during the admissions process. I found the advanced medical directives too detailed and too overwhelming to think about, so brought them home to look at. They, of course, kept getting set aside as each time I'd pick them up, I'd become overwhelmed, and set them aside again.

At each quarterly care plan meeting with the nursing home, the social worker would again prompt me to complete the Advanced Directives. Initially, when my mother was highly functional, there was little I would withhold as far as treatment; consequently, I found the Advanced Directives questions too detailed and did not want to make those decisions at that time.

About a year after Mom entered the nursing home, as her dementia progressed and her overall quality of life potential decreased, I realized I did not want her subjected to the drastic measures of resuscitation (e.g., CPR, defibrillation, etc.). I felt, if her heart stopped, she was at peace, and technically gone: there was no reason to put her through the pain and trauma of bringing her back when there was little quality of life potential to bring her back to. The experience would be painful, confusing and scary for her with no real benefit thereafter, so, I felt comfortable that in a full cardiac arrest situation, to let nature take its course and let her go peacefully. However, I still did not feel that I could complete the entire detailed Advanced Directives. I spoke with the social worker and learned that I could simply complete a DNR (Do Not Resuscitate) order rather than the entire Advanced Directives form. I opted to do that because that was the only scenario I felt comfortable with at that time. I also felt the Advanced Directives were not as critical; because, unlike a full cardiac arrest situation where there is no time for a decision (in the absence of a signed DNR, medical personnel are obligated to take full resuscitation measures), the Advanced Directive situations (e.g. artificial hydration and nutrition measures) allowed time for those decisions to be made at the time of need.

Knowing that signing a DNR was absolutely in Mom's best interests, the right thing to do, and what my mother would want, did not make doing so easy by any means. I was anxious and torn during the day and tossed and turned at night for the three days between making the decision and signing the document. And signing it did not immediately bring a peaceful resolve, so I spent another several days in anguish over this decision after the signing. There was this feeling that I was somehow killing (or aiding in the killing of) my mother. Intellectually I knew this was the right decision, but it took time to come to terms with it emotionally. This happened once I was able to understand (with some initial words from the social worker and some further research on Google) that resuscitation measures (from chest compressions to heart injections to defibrillation) were never intended to extend the life of terminally ill or elderly patients dying from natural causes that had little hope of any quality of life after resuscitation. These drastic measures were created to revive a patient who could be brought back, repaired if needed, and returned to a reasonable quality of life — not to remove the dignity of our final natural death and replace a peaceful passing with additional pain and confusion.

TESTED: Once I came to terms with this, I felt fairly peaceful and was able to let the new DNR drift to the back of my mind and not dwell on it. However, about a month after signing the DNR, I got a call from the nursing home about an hour after arriving home from visiting my mom (who was fine at the time I had left her) saying she was having some serious breathing issues and they were sending her to the ER. So, I raced to the hospital and met her in the ER. By this stage her dementia had progressed quite a bit. In addition to wanting to be with her, find out what was wrong, and oversee her care, I mostly was concerned that she would be frightened with the rapid transport, new environment, different people in and out, and overall commotion. The nursing home had sent her applicable paperwork with her; so, the ER doctor confirmed with me that my mother had an active DNR. I replied "Yes," but suddenly all the doubt rushed back in. In almost a panic, I began to think, *"Was it the right decision? Was it too soon? Would I really let her go if her heart stopped?"*

While attending my mom in the curtained ER examination room, a female patient was rushed into the adjacent room. As it happened, there was a slight gap where the curtains separating the two examining rooms met, so I had a clear view. Normally, I would have closed the curtain completely or not looked, but it all happened so quickly and I was not able to reach the curtain. I saw the woman first being slammed down on the exam table, then someone hopping on top of her and straddling to begin compressions and pounding on her chest. A few seconds later that action was replaced with needles into the heart and what seemed like endless attempts to resuscitate her with the defibrillator (the shock paddles), each time thrusting her body upwards several inches. What an awful and brutal procedure to watch. I finally received my peace of heart that I would never want my mother, in her current condition, to be subjected to that, only to possibly come back to finish her battle with Alzheimer's, with the added confusion of not understanding what happened or why she was now in so much pain (from the resuscitation).

Having the decision making authority as her *Health Care Proxy* was a Godsend because in this instance (and others) the decision was so mentally, emotionally, and physically taxing for me, I cannot fathom the added anxiety to obtain an HCP/POA through legal channels (without Mom's consent) would have caused me. I continued for a couple more years with just the DNR in place.

Advanced Directives: As my mother's condition continued to decline along with her quality of life potential, I came to realize that trips to the ER were more detrimental to her comfort than not going would be detrimental to her health.

Again, my constant goal was that she be as content and comfortable as possible with the best quality of life she was capable of achieving at any point in time. Trips to the ER were long, scary, and often unnecessary. I realized this one night when she had become very ill with the flu and a respiratory infection, and staff recommended that rather than transporting her to the ER they simply have the tests come to her. What? I never knew this was an option. I hesitantly agreed, and as I headed to the nursing home hoped I wasn't compromising her level of care. The "STAT" (immediate) orders were called in for blood work, EKG, and chest X-ray. Within an hour, each technician arrived one by one to administer their test. An IV was also started to ensure she was hydrated and to allow for fast administering should any drugs be needed. All this occurred within an hour of the phone order — all with Mom comfortably sleeping through most of it in her own room. Her only complaint was a few grunts when they rose her bed to a sitting position for the chest X-ray, then she went right back to sleep afterwards. When she was attended by staff (other than the mobile technicians) it was by staff she knew. There was no rapid transport, no sirens, no scary unfamiliar ER environment, and no strange staff in and out, poking and prodding. The icing on the cake was that all the test results were back in a couple of hours, so within three to four hours of making the phone call to order the tests we had the results; and all the while, Mom was comfortably sleeping in her bed, in her room, attended by the staff she knew. Prior experiences in the ER were never that fast, as she could lie there for hours before tests were given, and wait hours more before a doctor would come and discuss the results. Several times we were in the ER all night, not because she needed an admission, but simply because they were that slow. After this experience, I realized that in her current condition, and with a DNR, there was little that could be done in the ER that couldn't be done right there at the nursing home, in her bed and without commotion. So, I then took on the task of filling out the complete Advanced Directives form to ensure that Mom would never again be automatically transported to the ER. This was an easy decision because for any given incident, I could override that.

TESTED: Once again, I was tested on my decision. A month or so after having completed the Advanced Directives form, I got a call in the evening that my mother had had some sort of loss of consciousness episode and they thought she should be transported to the ER. I asked what her status was at that moment, and they said she was once again alert and unaware of the episode. I asked if she was comfortable. When they said yes, I instructed them to put her to bed, order whatever tests they wished to have done in her room, and said I'd be right there. I got an argument from the nurse on staff that evening as she preferred to send Mom out rather than attend her there, so I played the *"If you violate her advanced directives, expect to hear from my attorney"* card and she complied. When I arrived at the nursing home, my mother was sleeping comfortably, and soon the various technicians for the tests that were ordered came and went, and Mom was totally fine. The campus physician spoke to me and said if it was something serious, such as a silent heart attack, and I didn't send her to the ER, she could die. I asked what he thought could be done for her in the ER that couldn't be done in her room given her DNR and he said nothing really. He then agreed that it was better that she was more comfortable in her own room, but he had felt obligated to encourage me to send her. There was never a conclusive diagnosis, nor do I believe there would have been had she gone to the ER. I knew I had made the correct decision. Mom lived many more years without a repeat episode. But, even if she had passed away that night from natural causes, she would have been peaceful and comfortable, in her bed, and I knew it would have been okay if that had been her time to go.

7 Interacting With The Facility

Once Mom was a resident in a facility, my role as primary caregiver did not end, nor did it lessen. I suppose it could have had I chosen to become less involved, but that was simply not where I was in life and I wanted to ensure Mom got the best care available to her. So I was present at the facility on an almost daily basis, for visits with Mom, taking her out until the last years, and interacting with the management and staff to continually guide, adjust and nudge her quality of care as much as I could. I was fortunate to be in a facility where the management was truly interested in caregiving and willing to work with me, so it was easy for me to always begin any meeting on a positive note. However, I still recommend attempting this even if the management you are dealing with is not as helpful. You may find that beginning with a positive statement helps set the tone of the meeting and helps them let their defenses down, so they are able to work with you without feeling that they are on trial for something. I would usually begin by thanking them for the positive things in Mom's care, the facility, and aspects of the routine I thought they were doing well. I would praise the hands-on staff. And then I would say "There's so much you do here so well, but one thing I find that could use some improvement for my mom is . . ." — and then I'd begin the discussion about the issue for which I had called the meeting. I always let them know that

I did appreciate the 90% they did well and I wanted to work with them to help them improve on the areas that fell short. Sometimes that meant I extended myself more than I was required to, but it showed good faith on my part; and, in the end, my primary goal was to improve some situation in Mom's life.

So whether at meetings that I requested, a scheduled care plan meeting, or an impromptu barging into someone's office for a critical situation I felt could not wait for a routine meeting, I always tried to begin on a positive note, so I wasn't starting the confrontation as an enemy, but rather as a friend.

I was very fortunate that the facility my mother was in almost always met me halfway or more, no matter what level of management I sought out; and occasionally I was interacting with the highest onsite facility administrator, and once the corporate office. Another thing I did *almost* always was not to break hierarchy. If I could get results by simply chatting with her CNA then that's where the issue would stop: there was no reason to elevate it. Then the nursing supervisor, unit nurse manager and/or unit director (peers but one was medical management and the other was program management). Finally, I would walk into the facility administrator's office when necessary. Keeping this hierarchy accomplished two things. First, by resolving an issue at the lowest possible level, that person (such as a CNA) was able to correct an issue without being reported or written up for it and they greatly appreciated that. Second, it meant I complained fewer times to each management level in the hierarchy, so when I did go to the higher levels, I wasn't viewed as someone who was always complaining about something. Along those same lines, I also chose my battles carefully. There was rarely a visit when I couldn't find something to be improved upon if I looked; after all, this was my mother, so in my heart I wanted perfection. However, I knew to restrain that and only bring one or two issues at a time, and only when they affected my mother's comfort in some way. And that changed as her dementia progressed. Things that may have bothered Mom when she was highly functional and aware did not bother her later on because she was oblivious to them. So I made sure not to complain about small things that perhaps bothered me, but made no difference to my mother. I did witness other very devoted family members who hadn't caught on to that; so they were labeled cranks and chronic complainers and management often dismissed their complaints out of habit, sometimes not recognizing when there might have been a legitimate issue.

8 When And How The End Comes

Many Alzheimer patients die of something else (e.g. heart attack, stroke, or another unrelated cause) before reaching the terminal end of Alzheimer's disease. Some, like my mother, are healthy enough that they live through the entire duration of Alzheimer's and die from its effects. During the first few years that my mother was in the dementia unit, I observed the final weeks of several residents who went the full run of Alzheimer's. It wasn't long before I had categorized them in my mind into a few different scenarios – not an exact science of course, as each case is individual and not always textbook. The most common, and the one that I quickly decided was the scenario I hoped for when it was my mother's time, seemed to be the most natural, easiest on the patient, and the least emotional on the family because it was initiated by the patient. Also, because the patient was naturally giving the signals that it was time for the end, it seemed to be the most dignified for the patient. This scenario was that at some point, the patient would simply stop eating and drinking, refusing to accept any food or drink by mouth. Occasionally all at once, but often the eating would diminish and then stop altogether; then within a few days, liquids would be refused. At first, I thought these poor patients should be given IVs for hydration and at least a little nourishment. However, it's amazing how my perspective changed once I was routinely exposed to death and dying people.

I came to learn that when someone has a terminal illness or is at the natural end of their life, it is not in their best interest to take extraordinary or artificial measures to prolong life for those extra days or weeks, keeping them in discomfort or pain. Often the motivation to do so is selfish on our part as we do not want to lose them, but this is unfair to the patient if he or she is ready to pass on. I found this especially true after witnessing several lives ending in the scenario where the patient simply stopped taking nourishment. The more I observed this ending, the more natural and dignified it appeared to me. Now I'm not speaking of a patient who is not at the end of their terminal illness or natural life and is simply sick, such as with an intestinal virus that has left them dehydrated and too sick to eat. In that instance I would have given my mother an IV hydration if needed, to get over the few-day hump while she was fighting off the virus. I'm talking about when you know they have wound down, have little if any quality of life left, and are simply ready to go. The body may signal that by beginning to shut down, and part of that shutdown process is eating and drinking less, sleeping much more, and eventually refusing food and drink altogether.

a) The Last Days and Your Loved One

If you have notice of the end being near, the goal is to make your loved one's final days as comfortable and peaceful as possible. This can be achieved through a variety of things, including medications, music, a fan, and of course, your presence.

During the final few days of Mom's life, I put all of the above into place. I rotated her two favorite CDs (traditional Gospel hymns and more modern, but gentle, praise songs) so one of them was always playing, very softly. I brought in a small tabletop fan, set it across the room, and oscillated it around the bed (though not directly at her). I was told that circulating air can help a patient's breathing in the final days. The nursing home provided us with lemon glycerin swabs to clean and wet her mouth and lips periodically. I also brought some lip balm to keep her lips from drying and cracking. Each hour I would clean and wet her mouth with a lemon glycerin swab and apply the lip balm. Even though she appeared to be sleeping most times, she proved otherwise. I would always tell her what I was about to do, and when I got to the lip balm, I'd say that I was putting a little lipstick on her. Each time I finished running the lip balm over her lips she'd smack and rub her lips together, just as she always did when she applied lipstick throughout her life – that "girly-girl" was still in there, right until the end.

Additionally, I did my best to keep visitors to a minimum and their visits short, as each time people came to visit, Mom would become agitated. I tried to strike a balance between letting a few close relatives say their good-byes and keeping Mom peaceful, but my primary concern was Mom's comfort.

Our nurse practitioner prescribed three medications (morphine, Ativan, and something for nausea). The nausea medication was a patch that went behind her ear to prevent possible nausea from not eating. The morphine and Ativan were liquid which they could squirt into her mouth (not to be swallowed but to be absorbed in her mouth). These two were prescribed as needed, as frequent as once an hour, with me in control of when and how often they would be administered.

I allowed the patch to be placed behind her ear right away to be sure she was not nauseous. Knowing that Mom always had a very low tolerance for medications, particularly strong ones, I didn't want her to be over-medicated because the effects of that could make her feel sick. As long as she was comfortable, I also wanted her to have some awareness so she would know I was there and she could communicate (with expressions or simply squeezing my fingers) if she so chose. So her aides, the nurse, and I watched her carefully for signs of discomfort. For the first two days she was quite comfortable, so we only administered the nausea patch and a Tylenol suppository every three to four hours when they checked her for dryness and repositioned her.

When I arrived on the morning of what became her last day, there was a very noticeable difference from when I had left her late the night before. Her breathing, which had been strong, was now a bit labored and she seemed less comfortable, especially when her aide came in to check and reposition her. So with the nursing director's input, I made the decision to begin the morphine and Ativan — the morphine was for discomfort and the Ativan was to reduce anxiety and calm her breathing. Mom responded very well and I only needed to repeat those every three to four hours, about 20 minutes before her being repositioned, which seemed to be the times when she was in the most discomfort. It worked well, keeping Mom comfortable and peaceful, but still with times of being awake to know I was there with her.

I was fortunate that Mom passed quite peacefully in her sleep at 11:00 p.m., holding my two fingers as she always did.

b) The Last Days and You

Everyone reacts differently in an end-of-life situation. However you react will be normal for you, so don't judge yourself, simply go with it and do the best you can. The most important thing is to keep your focus on your loved one's comfort and peace.

I was quite numb and emotionless. From the moment the unit manager and I decided to accommodate Mom's refusal to eat or drink, my mission became ensuring that Mom's last days were the most comfortable they could be and that she felt loved and not alone. It is not uncommon for me in any stressful or difficult situation to automatically block off my emotions so I can deal logically with the situation. Then, when it is over, the built-up emotions flood in all at once and release. However, I was aware that I felt even more mechanical and detached than was normal for me while making decisions to ensure Mom's comfort. Although this was not my fault, nor was it wrong (it was simply how it affected me), this would come back to haunt me in the later stages of grief.

Several hours before my mother passed, one of her regular, very experienced aides told me to tell her it was okay for her to go, that I'd be okay. I wasn't sure about this — but when I was alone with Mom, at her bedside, with her holding my two fingers as she always did, it felt natural and right. Her eyes were closed and I wasn't sure if she was sleeping, even with her grasping my two fingers. Nor did I know, even if she was awake, if at this final stage of Alzheimer's where she had been non-communicative for so long if my words would have any meaning to her. But I told her that if Jesus, her mother or father, or Auntie Ellie came, it was okay for her to go with them. I said I would miss her, but I'd be okay and one day I would go to. Her breathing calmed down and she seemed more relaxed.

Once Mom passed, I was still numb, as the mission had not yet ended. I had a compulsion to ensure that I did not have to return to the nursing home the next day, with Mom now gone. Two days before, when Mom had gone to bed for the last time, I brought home everything I was going to take that I wouldn't need for her comfort for her last few days. Additionally, I brought bubble wrap and bags to package up her many framed artworks and personal effects that adorned the walls of her room. I left those up until after she passed, so if she opened her eyes at any time she would see her things on the walls and know she was in her familiar place. The nursing home offered to move her to a private room so she wouldn't be disturbed by her roommate, but I declined as I did not want her to be in a strange room in case she was at all aware.

God was good in answering my prayers of many years that Mom would pass peacefully at a time of her choosing, with me at her bedside. So many of those details could have gone awry for many reasons, and I am thankful that God scripted those last few days of Mom's life for us.

9 Grieving

Grieving is, of course, different for each person, and there is no right or wrong type or amount of grief. All feelings are valid and you may even experience seemingly conflicting emotions (loss vs. relief or guilt vs resentment, fear, anger, and a plethora of others). Some emotions will be concurrent; others will come and go throughout the grieving process. Whatever you are feeling, accept it as a valid feeling with no judgment attached and deal with each one, one at a time. It's okay to ask yourself why you think you have a certain emotion (especially if it's one you would not have expected), but try to do it objectively and do not label the emotion as good or bad. Whatever you are feeling, you may find that having been a Primary Caregiver will add a depth to the grieving process that you may not anticipate.

Personally, grieving for someone for whom I had been the caregiver over a 13-year period was far different than any other loss I'd experienced in my life. I was amazed at how much grief and emotions poured out beginning the day after my mother's passing. Given that it was a 13-year run with Alzheimer's and that she had been winding down her last six months, her death was something I assumed I would be completely prepared for. And especially after having been so numb during her last few days, I had thought it was because I was so prepared. But in hindsight, I think I was so detached because it was too emotional and that detachment allowed me to make rational decisions to ensure Mom's comfort in passing.

Beginning the day after her passing, and for the next week, the emotions came out in what seemed like an endless waterfall. I was able to hold up during the funeral preparations, but once I was home alone, they continually poured forth. Though I was shocked at the depth of grief I felt, I began to realize it was threefold (at least). First, of course, I had the loss of my mother, and second, the loss of my last link to that generation as she had survived all her siblings and my father and his sibling. But the third level was that I had gotten more and more attached to her during her last 13 years, first when she lived at home, and then when she went to the nursing home. During her first years in the nursing home, I went about five days a week, taking off two of the days my aunt went, so I knew she was seen by family every day. During the last several years when she declined to pureed food, I increased to six days a week. In her last 18 months, I often went seven days a week. I realized that when caring for someone on a daily basis, you develop a much deeper attachment to that person; this surprised me as we had always been close. But you simply become more invested in that person somehow. That person becomes a priority in your life as you adjust all other activities and relationships around them. They also become your focus and purpose in life. While caregiving drains much energy, it is also very fulfilling, putting into perspective what is important in life. Because it is the loss of all those things that contribute to the grief process, you may be surprised at the depth of grieving you will experience for someone after having been their caregiver.

The other thing I learned about grieving that surprised me was that the healing process was not linear, as it had been with every other loss I'd had throughout my life. Rather than the grief diminishing continuously over time, there were ups and downs and spikes and unexpected triggers on an otherwise seemingly better day. Just when I thought I had started to move on from the deep grieving stage, I'd see an item in the grocery store that I used to buy specifically for Mom, and it would trigger a major grief moment — sometimes causing me to just leave the store without buying anything. There was a full year of that before I leveled off and only had occasional, mild grief spikes beyond whatever level I was at.

I think forgetting was the most difficult for me, both in that I missed the vivid memories and had sadness as those emotions faded. For many months after Mom's passing when I'd get up each day I'd close my eyes and remember going to feed her breakfast — and I could feel her presence, smell her scent, and feel her grasping my fingers, as if the moment was real. As time went on, those feelings and emotions gradually faded, leaving the memories: but they were much less vivid, less real, and less in-the-moment, experiences.

One thing that took the longest for me to come to terms with was my emotional detachment during her last few days. I would get times of deep grief, wondering if due to my detachment my mother did not feel loved in her last few days, but rather felt like an inanimate object I was going through the motions with. But as time passed, the actual memories of those blurred last days came into perspective. I realized that when I was at her bedside and she was holding my two fingers, I was always compassionate and loving both in speech and tasks as I attended to her needs. This was my personal grief issue, but I wanted to share this because in speaking with others who lost their loved around the same time Mom passed, I found each caregiver seemed to have their own personal grief issue. One was that she wasn't there at the moment her loved one passed. Of course it is not always possible to be at the bedside at the time of passing. While this woman logically knew that, it was still her personal grief issue. It seemed that since as caregivers we strived to give the very best care, we each had an issue for which we worried our efforts may have fallen short — and that became our personal grief issue. If you find yourself with one, you likely will eventually put it into perspective, but not necessarily early on.

Epilogue:
Caring for the Caregiver

Caregiving for the Caregiver could be a book in and of itself, so my brief coverage of this topic at the end is not meant to suggest that it is unimportant, but rather that the purpose of this book is to discuss issues and solutions with dementia patient care, not caregiver care. However, it is because of the great importance of this related topic that I decided this book would be incomplete without at least a mention.

For most caregivers, taking care of themselves is indeed an afterthought as they pour their attention and energy into the care of their loved one, often at the expense of their own well-being. This isn't much different than a parent who puts the care of their child before their own care. And just as a child's needs may seem endless, leaving little time and attention for the parent's needs, so too the needs of the dementia patient often leave little time for the caregiver's self-care — at least from the caregiver's perspective.

I will dispense with a lecture on how a caregiver can't give the best care if he or she is depleted physically, mentally, and emotionally because caregivers know this, and will likely be repeatedly reminded of this truth by well-meaning people around them. But, as I did, many caregivers will ignore this all too sound advice and continue to neglect their own well-being for the care of their loved one.

In a perfect scenario, a caregiver would ensure that their own care and well-being are always sufficient. However, it would be disingenuous of me to give the impression that I came even close to that: because I did not. My primary concern was my mother's care and I usually put my well-being on the back burner. I'm not recommending or even excusing this practice, but being a realist, I am acknowledging that the norm for caregivers leans more toward neglecting themselves than maintaining the proper care they need and deserve.

At some point, you may need to accept that the quality of your visits is as important as the quantity. Watch for your limits as they affect your loved one and adjust accordingly to achieve a balance between quantity and quality. There was a point at which I realized that in a completely depleted state, being with my mother was more negative for her than positive. After my Aunt Ellie (who had visited Mom three times a week) became ill and passed away, I increased my visits from five days a week to seven. I had been used to Mom being seen and fed a meal by family every day, and I didn't want to her lose that. After several weeks of going every day with no time to rejuvenate or regroup, I became completely burnt out.

And that run down state affected my interactions with my mother. I realized I was suddenly less interested and less engaging — eager to get through her meal, which made me less patient. We were both getting less from the visit and it became clear to me that I needed to stop visiting Mom one day a week to clear my head. I had to accept that she'd be fine for a day without me. Would she eat less that day? Yes. Would she be less engaged, less talked to, and less entertained that day? Most Definitely. But she would be fine overall.

I decided to take Thursdays off since it was my last dinner visit for the week and Fridays began my breakfast visits. So in reality, I was only postponing my visit by about 15 hours, from Thursday night dinner to Friday morning breakfast. And some amazing things happened once I began to take that one day a week off from visiting Mom, changing my initial concern of being absent to satisfaction in how both Mom and I reacted.

First, and not surprisingly, I was refreshed, clear-headed, and couldn't wait to get to Mom's on Friday mornings, both because I'd had time to regroup and also that I had time to miss her. More surprising was Mom's reaction to me on Friday mornings. After my aunt's health forced her to stop visiting, my mother deeply missed her sister. She seemed to have grown tired of seeing my face every day instead of the alternating visits by my aunt and me that she had been accustomed to for so many years. But once I began skipping Thursday visits, Mom was all smiles and so happy to see me on Friday mornings — she now had a chance to miss me!

The last thought I'll offer on *Caring for the Caregiver* is that it needs to continue after your loved one passes on and your caregiver duties have ended. Throughout, and especially toward the latter stages of grieving, you will need to begin to replace all that time you had dedicated to your loved one with other endeavors for yourself. For some, this may happen naturally. However, oftentimes, as a caregiver you may have drifted away from social relationships and activities due to having devoted so much time to your loved one. Sometimes it may take a conscious and planned effort to re-establish friendships and rebuild your life.

Made in the USA
Columbia, SC
09 March 2020